# Thinner and Healthy Living

## A Complete Guide To Achieving Your Perfect Body Image

Jessica Bailey

# Copyright

- Table Of Contents

INTRODUCTION

CHAPTER ONE

Goal Setting For Weight Management

CHAPTER TWO

The Reason Goals Are Important in Weight

Loss

CHAPTER THREE

The Reason Goals Are Important In Weight

Management

CHAPTER FOUR

The Reason Goals Are Important In Body

Image

# INTRODUCTION

Weight loss is one of the main concerns of public health officials who care about maintaining a good and better life. They focus on this area of work so that they can easily control and monitor the condition of anyone who needs support, medication and treatment so that these people can overcome their difficulties in their feeding program. The concept of this book is to make people aware of why they need to be aware of their weight and how to prevent diseases that may appear soon simply because they neglected their unhealthy situation.

There are countless reasons why obese or

overweight people try to lose weight. Some want to be healthier, feel and look better, while others want more energy to do their daily tasks.

Whatever the reason, healthy weight management and successful weight loss depend on reasonable goals and expectations. When you set goals, it's not impossible to reach them and have a chance to maintain your weight.

Anyone can lose weight effectively. Get all the information you need here.

Chapter One

# Goal Setting For Weight Management

Publications are the first thing government

agencies produce to effectively convey their important communication to the public; to be healthy with the help of weight loss operations. They continue to produce tools that can help them reach people who are ignorant of their situation. These publications also contain food-related information and practices that people can follow to promote healthier living. In this way, numerous people will no longer know which specific weight loss operation processes are preferred for their requirements.

Weight loss is a term that's on numerous people's minds. Some need it for medical reasons and others for body image purposes. While there are numerous results available in a moment's request and advice can be set up over the internet, achieving weight loss successfully is a different matter.

People struggle to lose weight substantially because of wrong prospects and misguidance due to different product marketing. Before you rush and start on your weight loss plan, wait to consider some weight loss basics first.

As for the focus of people who in no way stop trying to overcome the cause and effect of poor weight loss operation, people who now continue to do their best their way will no longer have difficulty achieving results. more recommended than they've always wanted. When they achieve these results, they're now suitable to view their life prospects in a more positive light, which is the main reason they can be productive as healthy people

# Chapter Two

# The Reason Goals Are Important In Weight Loss

The importance of weight loss management is now recognized as a top priority by healthcare providers and government agencies. Since health is a concern, there is a great chance that many people will solve their problems now, when the time comes when they are aware of how to live a healthier life.

Goals and their meaning

When you perform each of these tasks in sequence, you foster the possibility of people living longer while prospering.

Consequently, it is better to know the following important facts about weight loss management that will help you realize how valuable it is to own.

Diabetes is considered one of the main diseases of young and old people. As you know, diabetes causes many difficulties in life if it is not prevented and treated properly. With the presence of weight loss management, there is a definite chance that people can avoid the possibility of developing diabetes, which can cause many serious and incurable diseases.

Never neglect this type of condition if you

have it, as it can weaken you as a person in terms of declining health.

Another thing that makes weight loss management important is that it can help blood circulate properly in your body's system. The regular supply and circulation of blood, including the balance of its flow and existence, will develop positive results that can rid you of diseases and illnesses. Weight loss management can also help maintain your glucose levels, which prevents your body from losing its strong immune system. With the help of weight loss management, you will no longer have any difficulty in creating healthy cells in your body.

As long as you practice and support healthy living that comes with weight loss management, you will never lose your confidence as a person. Many obese people do not want to go shopping or participate in other activities because of their size and health. It is better to move to maintain and prevent this type of situation. Along with weight loss management, you now have the assurance of being fit and efficient in daily tasks and activities.

Cholesterol, blood pressure and any other type of cardiovascular disease can only be controlled and prevented by controlling weight loss. If you exercise every day, you can better defend yourself against these diseases, which are considered one of the reasons why a person cannot adequately complete all the tasks assigned to them during the day. Being unhealthy is not an option, especially when you have a family that relies on strength and confidence that can see you through it.

# Chapter Three

# The Reason Goals Are Important In Maintaining Weight

Compelling reasons are often the reason to think about a healthy and active life. With the support of a weight maintenance system, you, as a person who aspires to a life fit to face the various challenges of life, especially when it comes to the existence of diseases and illnesses, will no longer have problems with your plans.

Weight maintenance systems

Weight Maintenance Systems will give you results that are proud to be endorsed and recommended to others. It is beneficial to get the results that come from this system so that you can avoid the difficulty of living a happy and content life.

Calories in the body, if not balanced, can bring weakness to the body. Too much of anything is always bad and useless. So when you have a calorie count that exceeds your body's ability to recover, it's time to embark on a weight maintenance program. Maintaining your body weight like an average person can save you calories. A healthy and balanced eating habit will help make your dietary goals more successful and truly achievable.

Fiber helps the body's system to function properly. It also generates energy that can help improve your work, leading to good performance. A weight maintenance system is also important when considering the presence of fiber, as this is a factor that can eliminate the possibility of disease development. Fiber is also helpful for a person to be fully conditioned every day. When you get that result from fiber, you don't have to worry about how to maintain good shape and weight.

A body with a balanced and clean fluid composition is also important for maintaining weight composition.

Water helps a person feel full from time to time, which means you may now lose your appetite for unhealthy foods. Water is also good for the digestive system as it prevents the digestive process from becoming difficult. The ease of digestion helps nutrients from food reach every potential part of your body for a strong and healthy life. Finally, water is invaluable when it comes to maintaining the coolness and balance of your body's fluid and sweat systems.

Physical activity of the body increases your metabolism, which is great for the productivity of your life. As a result, you can now achieve many things with the help of a weight maintenance system that was previously unparalleled. In addition, it can also increase your metabolism rate, which is considered to be a great help for your body to resist diseases. Now it is possible to burn fat in an effortless process.

# Chapter Four

## The Reason Goals Are Important In Body Image

Indeed, body image can affect the way you live your life and the tasks you have to do for other people every day. Possessing good curves and muscles that are strong helps a person to perform the work and operations in his job better because these factors increase his self-confidence. It is also a fact that body image influences other people's impression that they are strangers. Coupled with a healthy and fit lifestyle, you can easily achieve the body image that many people dream of.

Body image is important

With a good body curve that is shapely and healthy at the same time, you will feel great every day. Since the function of body image is to reveal your outer beauty, people will notice your truly disciplined and responsible lifestyle. In addition to these benefits, you can now achieve the best self-confidence, self-acceptance, and self-esteem, which is helpful for your personality development. You can also prevent tendencies that lead to eating habits and mood disorders that are unhealthy since they affect the person's psychological system and can make them more depressed.

Your mind and body are always connected in every way, in this case, with a good body structure, there is a great chance that you too can have good prospects in life. So when people think that you are not physically fit, it can also affect your mind. But never be disappointed by this, it is better to solve the problem with the help of a healthy and balanced diet accompanied by regular exercise. This lifestyle will help you realize the importance of your body image.

The poor bodies could experience a lot of discrimination and other related insults that can damage their confidence and self-esteem. It is good that you can accept your true self so that you never feel insecure when other people receive good impressions from the public. That way, even if you're not perfect, you can see your worth as a person. You can also generate standards that

allow more positive thoughts to arise that produce worthwhile and genuinely satisfying actions such as wellness. Appreciating yourself is a good thing that can help a person achieve his life plans. A healthy body encourages better thinking because it can give you stable enough thoughts for work and tasks that require immediate and satisfying solutions. Stable emotions and mental systems will prevent you from viewing things in life as negative. In this case, it is possible to reduce the probability of feeling depressed and the presence of anxiety, since these factors are the main reasons why a person thinks negatively about life.

# Chapter Five

# Tips For Setting Goals For Eating Right

Eating healthy, balanced meals is one of the best ways to live longer and richer. The moment you start living well, especially eating well, there's no way you can't feel good about yourself and your outward appearance. Many beneficial effects are only possible if you start leading this lifestyle. Never underestimate the power of this system and the nutritional structure that makes up this very healthy approach, as it will give you the confidence to achieve a strong and positive feeling of well-being.

How to eat well

Whole grains are one of the best types of foods to add to your diet plan. Its abundance in the market can also be added to your plan since you will never have a problem finding these products. Another thing is that whole grains can be accompanied by different types of food such as vegetables and fruits and even milk; There are many ways to consume this food. The importance of whole grains in your body is that they can provide the natural nutrients necessary for all the energy your system needs each day. A variety of whole grains can also give you more flexibility when eating these healthy foods.

Vegetables are well known for having good effects on the body, but sometimes people find it difficult to consume them because of their structure and appearance. That's the best thing about vegetables because, just like fruits, you can now drink them through mixed systems. Another thing that will surprise you about this food is that it can be eaten raw. You just have to clean it properly. Incorporating vegetables into your diet plans can help to properly neutralize the foods you eat every day. It can also cleanse your body system as it contains natural nutrients that cleanse your digestive system and other related factors.

Fruit is also considered a common food

eaten by people who want to have good eating habits. As you know, fruits are composed of various vitamins and minerals that build immunity so that the body can resist diseases and illnesses. They can also refresh the body to make it more alive. The fruits also serve as a natural remedy that can make your skin look more attractive and fresh. As long as you're consuming fruit, there's no way you can get a natural approach to proper nutrition.

It goes without saying to maintain a consistent diet on a low-fat system. If you want to fry, only use non-stick pans so that you stop using oil that contains a lot of fat. Start your morning with oatmeal, in a bowl, to give you all the benefits you need for the day. Limit your intake of sweet foods and avoid smoking. These are some of the details

that can help you achieve nutritional
success.

# Chapter Six

# Tips For Setting Goals For Exercise

To achieve the desired training effects, you must be motivated, committed, and disciplined to meet and achieve your goals. Yes, it is difficult because you have many commitments that have to be done every day. However, since you want to achieve these things, you should consider healthily approaching these tasks.

Practice target pointer

It is always good for a specific body system to move and work with precision so that you can live a healthy life in all aspects. To get the best results from this plan, you need to stay focused and fight for your goals.

The concrete objectives are really important to be visualized as soon as possible. In this way, you can avoid factors that could potentially interfere with your plans. Specific goals can also help you stay on track, as long as you stick to the plan, you're never in a failed state. You can also narrow down the reasons why you need to change your exercise program. Maintaining yourself and staying on track can give you the confidence to achieve your plan and goals. Measurable goals are also important to achieve. There is a good chance that knowing how to monitor your trades will make you aware of where you stand regarding your training status. As long as you implement such a system, you will no longer have trouble controlling your zeal which sometimes leads to accidents. Stopping and not exceeding the limit of your body is a great advantage in maintaining a good balance of your body's performance. Customizable goals are also helpful in making you feel good about the activities you do. Now you can adapt to different challenges, so the obstacles will never affect you.

Lifestyle. This is a very effective system to train your body without suffering injuries from hardcore learning. This process will also help you to be more flexible in every way. Because these destinations are considered flexible, you can easily reroute your route without getting lost.

An action-oriented goal refers to the application of exercises that cover your overall plan for reaching your healthy living goals.

In terms of realistic goals, this practice focuses on how to implement serious and rigorous training programs that truly lead to good body structure. Realizing and setting this goal will generate more power and motivation in your practice.

Time-based goals are specific plans that focus on your availability to exercise. Since you always have a busy work schedule, you must set a day that is focused on your training, which will never affect the process you need to do that day.

# Chapter Seven

## Tips For Setting Goals For Body Image

If you have decided to stay healthy by maintaining a body image that is truly beneficial to all, then your decision is truly a glimpse into the future and a better outlook in life. As is well known, being fit and sexy at the same time means plenty of chances and chances to stand out, not only through your outward appearance but also through your disciplined personality, which successful people commonly have. Now it is possible to grant you multiple credits for working with this technique to improve the state of your body image.

Body image goals

Lasting relationships can be achieved as long as you maintain your beauty inside and out. As an advice, it is good to have inspiration and motivation to carry out this act of extra healthy life. You can look for reasons like work, family and love life, and even problems with friends and relationships. It is a well-known fact that people only accept you based on first impressions, and, indeed, they cannot appreciate you as a person at first glance. This is just one motivating example that will help you immediately see how important body image is in the public eye.

Work habits require a lot of effort and energy. This reason can serve as a motivation for you to live a healthier life while having a great body. As long as you exercise and eat the right kinds of food, you can create positive systems for your body, such as intelligence and energy. As a result, you no longer need to worry about the results and achievements that will come soon after your efficient and effective work, accompanied by a good amount of encouragement and motivation.

Relationships will never have a good foundation if both partners do not have the motivation to become good people in terms of external and internal appearance. It is better to be aware of how to become a good person and that this also affects the way you encounter the outside world. Body image can also be one of the biggest motivators for a relationship to grow stronger.

Foundation, endowment. Yes, love is more important, but maintaining a respectable appearance can create more passion in love. Body image can be more beneficial because it can push people in a relationship into a more passionate state of romance when making love, which is very healthy for love, connection, and communication.

Your family, especially your children, need your time and effort when the day comes to an end after long and hectic hours. In this case, becoming more energetic is a motivation for you, since your work is not the only thing that requires your full attention. It is best to encourage a healthy lifestyle through exercise to promote the beneficial effects for your family that only a good body image can bring.

## Chapter Eight

## How To Stick To The Weight Loss Goals You Have Set

Sticking to your plans is beneficial when you are seriously dependent on achieving your goals. Through a healthy lifestyle, there is also a great chance to live a prosperous and comfortable life. So when the time comes when you decide to start exercising with your weight loss goals, you should never stop trying and practising the system that can offer you lifelong opportunities. It is also possible to gain many benefits by concentrating your time and dedication on making your weight satisfactory not only in other people's eyes but also to improve your health and life.

Tips to keep it up


To have a good focus on your weight loss goal plans, you must first write down all your reasons, specific practices, and how and when you will do those diets and exercises. Writing these things down gives you a head start and doesn't throw you off course. In this way, you can also check your achievements every time you practice your healthy hobby. Because you write down all of your plans, you also have more flexibility in case you miss parts.

Realize your objective as realistic; in other words, make sure you don't sacrifice too much. It is better to imagine things that can happen soon because anticipation will never lead to depression. Focusing on these achievable weight loss benefits will help you avoid stress.

# Chapter Nine

## How To Stick To The Weight Maintenance Goals You've Set For Yourself

Many ways can help you reach and maintain the weight loss goals you've set for yourself. But more often than not, these plans are difficult to implement in terms of reaching your goals. Consequently, there are additional actions that need to be taken along with your plans. These practices can help make your established plans beautiful and safe. Consequently, these supplements have proven their effectiveness in all conditions of the body structure.

Stick to your goals

Sleeping 7 to 8 hours is one of the healthy ways to fulfil your plans. As long as you get full hours of sleep, there's a good chance you'll get enough energy to reach your goals. Another benefit you can get from sleeping through the night is the focus your mind needs to do a better job. If you practice this particular act, there is no way you will fail in your plans. Consequently, you will never feel exhausted so quickly as you will have the energy you need before and after work hours.

Another factor that can help you achieve your goals is the presence of people who give you reasons to go ahead with your plans and goals. Make sure they don't affect your activities that make your plans invisible, which is very insignificant. Highly influential people often offer activities that are unhealthy and can ruin your healthy lifestyle. The perfect partners for your goals are those who can share knowledge and practices with you.

You can promote these plans to your friends and family. As long as you share your goals in these healthy practices with them, there's no way you won't find an interested person to accompany you in each of your workouts. This factor can also help you avoid people who can easily influence and ruin your plans. Have dinner with your friends and family, so you can find out about your fitness plans and with whom

You know, maybe some of them are already doing this salutary act, which is very suggestive.

Eating enough food is beneficial as it provides you with nutrients, vitamins and minerals that are good for your energy, and mental and emotional needs. In this way, you will never lose the strength that can keep you energized and save you from complete exhaustion. Plus, you won't feel hungry after every training session you participate in. When you lose fat, you can now easily replace it with foods that provide you with nutrients.

# Chapter Ten

## All The Good That Comes Out Of Great Goal Setting

The results are achievable and of course can be done in a short time if you are dedicated, focused on the procedures and always looking forward to a better tomorrow and the positive results of perseverance. While there are major roadblocks that may force you to give up trying, there are still numerous reasons and outcomes that will help you envision things that can keep you going and keep your plans on track. Along with these reasons, you will never have to face any difficulties as long as you are responsible for carrying out your goals. As a result, you can now achieve the most positive result that you have been looking for from the very beginning.

The advantages

Big plans seem out of reach, but if you have the perseverance to do them, there is nothing impossible in the process that you have to overcome and practice almost every day. Although there are times when you feel exhausted and stressed with your goals, you think that positive results, skills, knowledge and abilities only increase the limit, helping you to achieve the tasks you need to do.

Most of the time, there are vague goals, especially when you just start the task. But never give up, along with carrying out your plans, in the process of educating yourself and raising awareness, there is a great opportunity for you to make those goals visible and achievable. As a result, you can now have your goals well established and recorded on your organizational chart. This process will help you not to be confused about your training days compared to the next program you follow. This program is planned by professional fitness trainers. Don't worry as they will help you to be flexible about schedules.

Action plans become more productive and effective the more you work with your plan; This is a proven fact and a tried and tested system that is being done by many people concerned with the same goals as you. Never stop fighting for your goal and you will never regret the result obtained after each session. As you continue, you will gradually find that your lifestyle and body shape will change.

# Chapter Eleven

# Weight Loss Resolutions Basics

Losing weight is the term that comes to mind for many people. Some need it for medical reasons and others for cosmetic reasons.

While there are many solutions available on the market today and advice can be easily found on the internet, achieving weight loss goals is another matter entirely. People struggle to lose weight mainly due to false expectations and deception due to the marketing of different products.

Before you rush off and start your weight loss plan, first consider the basics of weight loss.

The basics of weight loss.

Losing pounds is one aspect of effective and successful weight loss. This is the basic idea that everyone can identify with. It can also be measured to achieve visible results. The words "weight loss" convey these ideas.

Losing weight revolves around several important aspects, including
Restore and improve your health, stay on track to achieve all your weight loss goals, and transform and maintain a leaner body. For you to successfully lose weight, you must follow the basic principles of weight

loss. These include the following:

Decrease

stay motivated

muscle development

For you to be successful, you have to remember to go the extra mile as there are no shortcuts to shed unwanted pounds.

Lose fat: diets can help you

A proper and healthy balanced diet is important for weight loss. Choose and follow a diet that is high in fibre and protein and low in refined carbohydrates.

Once you increase your fibre and protein intake, you will gradually lose weight and build strong muscles. When you eat fewer refined carbohydrates, you also get rid of the calorie buildup that isn't providing your body with the nutrients it needs.

Build Muscle: Do Some Workouts

Building muscle can help with weight loss. This is because fat is burned to give you the proper energy your muscles need to stay alive. It is interesting to note that a pound of fat only requires three calories to function, while a pound of muscle requires 75 to 150 calories per day. Therefore, if you want to see results while losing weight, you must exercise.

You can consider any exercise or training. However, anaerobic and aerobic exercise is essential to make your body work harder. For best results, change up your exercise routines to keep your body stimulated.

Some consider weight loss programs just for exercise. There are even others who sign up for a physical education class. You don't have to spend a lot of money when you exercise. You can train at home. Just select the exercises that do not require fitness equipment.

If you exercise, take it seriously and stick to your plan. Learn to be motivated. Exercise regularly with consistency and

Commitment is essential. Don't make mistakes and expect quick results like most people. You should keep in mind that it also takes time to see results.

Stay motivated

It is important to accept that weight loss does not happen quickly. Losing weight is a journey that requires you to monitor your progress. This way you can see results and at the same time be motivated with your plan.

Losing weight can be easy for some because they use magic pills. However, if you want to improve your overall health and maintain a healthy weight, stay motivated and keep going because you can make a difference.

# Chapter Twelve

## Use Walks For Exercise

Anyone can lose weight depending on the intensity and duration of the walk, as well as their diet. That is why many experts advise overweight people to walk as it can be a big part of their weight loss process. However, this does not mean that you have to give up a healthy and balanced diet. You must continue to stick to your weight loss plan. Walking is only an advantage for those who want to see results in a short time.

Walking as a bonus to your weight loss process

Some people say that physical activity like walking is not important when trying to lose weight. But the truth is that walking to lose weight can help you get the results you want.

If you consider adding 30 minutes of brisk walking to your daily activity, you would burn about 150 calories a day. For you to lose a pound each week, you need to get rid of 500 calories every day. The more time you spend walking and the faster your pace, the more calories you'll naturally burn.

To be successful at walking weight loss, you need to keep your exercise intensity at a vigorous or moderate level. When it comes to losing weight, the more you walk or the harder you walk, the more calories you burn. However, you should keep in mind that balance is essential.

If you are new to physical activity and regular exercise, you can start with a low intensity and gradually increase it. After successfully losing weight, you should not remove walking exercises from your daily routine, as this will help you maintain your weight. Studies have shown that people who maintain their weight long-term always consider regular walking. So go ahead and follow a healthy and balanced diet.

Guide to using the walk to lose weight

As mentioned above, walking alone will not help you successfully lose weight. You should still consider a healthy diet, as it can help you achieve all your weight loss goals.

Most people trying to lose weight find it difficult to stay on track. This guide will motivate you to lose weight.

watch your diet

The best key to avoiding overeating is to stay on top of what you're eating. It may seem like a simple task, but managing nutrition can be challenging. If you don't want to ruin your weight loss goals, keep track of what you eat or drink. It may also be a good idea to keep track of the calories in your food. By doing this you can maintain a healthy weight.

## Measure your walks

There are several ways to monitor your walks or the distance traveled. Distance tracking allows you to compare routes and can help you increase your distance, which also helps you burn more calories, which is crucial when walking to lose extra pounds.

## Keep a running record

Keeping a running log is just as important as keeping a diet log. This will help you stay motivated while you lose weight. Other than that, your walking log allows you to track your progress as you gradually increase the intensity of your walks.

# Chapter Thirteen

## Use Fruits Rich in Vitamin C

Recent studies suggest that if you eat more fresh citrus fruits and some vegetables and fruits rich in vitamin C, you will have more success in your weight loss. This doesn't mean that vitamin C is the new wonder weight-loss drug, but experts have found that taking too little of the vitamin can make it difficult to lose weight.

More information about vitamin C

Vitamin C doesn't just help with colds. If you need to lose weight for whatever reason, this vitamin can help you. Did you know that fruits rich in vitamin C can make you burn more fat?

What is vitamin C?

Vitamin C is also known as ascorbic acid. It is a water-soluble vitamin with an antioxidant function in the body. This simply means that it neutralizes free radicals that can damage cells.

Vitamins that are soluble in water are not stored in the body. Therefore, you should consider having a fresh supply every day. Otherwise, you risk developing a deficiency that can lead to health problems over time.

Unfortunately, the body can't make vitamin C. So it's important to make sure you're getting enough of this nutrient.

Vitamin C and weight loss.
If you are considering juice recipes for weight loss, you will get results if you include fruits rich in vitamin C.

Researchers are looking for vitamin C-rich fruits and vegetables that may increase fat burning during exercise. So eat some and use it in your juice recipes.

You can consider any fruit that is rich in vitamin C. If you have no idea which one is best for your weight loss needs, ask the experts for help. Also, if you have allergies to some fruits, you'd better consult your

doctor and ask for advice on the right fruits
to use.

# Chapter Fourteen

## Swap Trans Fats For Healthier Fats

For several years, doctors and nutritionists have preached that a low-fat diet is the best key to successful weight loss, preventing health problems, and controlling cholesterol levels.

Because of this, you must have ideas on how to replace trans fats (bad fats) with healthier fats. This is because bad fats can increase your health risks, while good fats can protect your overall health. The healthiest fats are important for emotional and physical health.

Eliminate trans fats from your diet

Trans fats are normal fat molecules that have been twisted and misshapen during a process called hydrogenation. In this process, liquid vegetable oil is combined with hydrogen gas and heated. In part, vegetable oils that are hydrogenated become less perishable and more stable, which is good for all food producers and not good for you, especially if you're at a healthy weight.

Trans fats are not healthy. Even a small amount is not healthy. The reason is that these fats contribute to several major health problems like cancer and heart disease.

Sources of trans fat

When it comes to trans fats, many think of margarine. Well, there are indeed several kinds of margarine that are loaded with these fats. However, the main source of trans fat in the Western diet is commercially prepared snack foods and baked goods.

Baked goods such as crackers, pizza dough, cookies, muffins, pie crusts and other bread, including hot dogs or hamburger buns. Snacks - Corn, candy, tortilla chips, potatoes, microwave or packaged popcorn. Fried foods: French fries, chicken nuggets, hard tacos, doughnuts, and fried chicken.

Pre-mixed products like pancake or cake mix, or chocolate drink mix.

Solid fats or semi solid, vegetable shortening or stick margarine.

Be a trans fat detective

When shopping for your monthly or weekly groceries, always read the labels and check the ingredients for trans fats. Some foods do not have a trans fat label, their ingredients may be suspect.

When shopping for margarine, choose versions like soft-tub and make sure products contain zero grams of this bad fat. If you are used to eating out, skip cookies, some baked goods, and fried foods. Unless your chosen restaurant does not use trans fats in the preparation of their meals, avoid these foods. Also, ask the person at the counter or the server what kind of oil is used to cook the food. If they use trans fat, you can ask them to prepare your dishes with olive oil.

If you want to successfully get rid of trans fats, one of the things you need to do is avoid fast food. Most states do not have labelling requirements for fast food. This can be advertised as cholesterol-free when the food is cooked in vegetable oil.

How to choose healthy fats

With so many sources of dietary fat, the choices can be confusing. But the bottom line is the good fats that give you tons of health and weight loss benefits.

If you're concerned about your heart health or your weight, instead of avoiding fats in your diet, try replacing the bad fats, like trans fats, with healthier fats. That just means replacing some of your meat with legumes and beans with the use of olive oil.

Eliminate trans fats from your diet. Whenever you go to a grocery store, always check the labels to find out how much trans fat is in what you are about to eat. Also, limit fast food.

Limit or try to avoid your intake of bad fats or saturated fats. You can limit saturated fat by cutting back on full fat dairy and red meat. The best alternatives to red meat are fish, beans, nuts, and if possible, fish. Also, switch to low fat versions of milk or full fat dairy products.

Consider eating omega-3s every day. The best sources of omega-3s are walnuts, fish, canola oil, soybean oil, ground flaxseed, and flaxseed oil.

How much fat is too much?

This depends on your current weight, lifestyle, age, and your health, all these will determine the amount of fat that is too much to maintain a healthy weight Condition. So if you're not sure how to measure your fat intake, talk to some experts or set your fat limit. You can't limit yourself to this, but you will also gradually reduce the bad fats without having to consider other avenues. Plus, this can put you on track to eating healthier fats.

Trans fats aren't just one of the bad fats to avoid when trying to lose weight. Saturated fat is also a type of fat found in various animal products. By reducing this bad fat, you can also achieve your weight loss goals effectively.

# Chapter Fifteen

# Reprogram Your Mind about Portion Sizes

When it comes to losing weight, it's important to eat the right serving size. However, many people trying to lose weight find it difficult to control their food portion sizes. Well, it's very difficult at first. But once you learn to control it, you can make some changes to your diet, and you can look at food portions as a tool for successful weight loss and healthier eating.

It can be impossible to measure every bite that passes your lips. However, it's a good idea to start measuring drinks and food until you feel like you're considering the correct portion sizes for weight loss.

With millions of foods out there, you might be surprised that a serving or two can make all the difference. So learn to reschedule your portion sizes, as it can play a huge role in weight loss.

Understanding portion sizes

People often equate portion sizes with the number of certain foods that are placed on their plates, just like in restaurants. Unfortunately, these are not serving sizes. Most of the time, the portions served do not reflect the actual serving size. That's why some find it difficult to control portion sizes.

Many people do not usually measure their food, even when they are at home. They usually guess what a serving of food is. Because of this, some do not understand the importance of true serving size.

To learn more about serving sizes, try measuring the serving size of your food. You won't be able to control your calorie intake this way, but you will also learn to control your portion sizes.

A general rule of thumb when portioning your plate

There are several ways to control portions.

Some of these are the following:

The size of a baseball or a woman's fist is equal to one serving of fruits and vegetables. A rounded handful equals about 1/2 cup of cooked pasta or rice.

The platform size is about three ounces of meat, which is a common serving size. The large egg or golf ball is about the same size as a quarter cup of walnuts. A computer mouse is about the size of a small potato.

Aside from the methods mentioned, measuring is still considered the best way to ensure you're eating the correct serving size. In the meantime, once you've measured your food, you can ensure you're getting the correct serving size.

If you're not sure you have the right size, try putting less on your plate. Then when you're hungry, have a second half serving just to be safe.

# Chapter Sixteen

## Change Your Mind About Salt and Use Fresh Herbs

Salt doesn't beget or cause your body to lose or gain fat. Salt has no calories. still, consuming large  quantities of  salt can beget or cause temporary weight gain. This is because salt causes your body to retain redundant water.

On the other hand, if you eat  lower salt, your body may lose some weight because your body is getting  relieved of water.

 It's  intriguing to note that almost all of the

crash diets that show rapid weight loss are grounded on foods with no or low salt content, still this doesn't mean that you're going to  exclude salt from your diet fully but if you want to see instant results, why not use fresh herbs rather than salt, In this way, you can't only lose weight but also have a healthier weight.

Why should you change your mind about salt?
 Although salt  is an essential part of the diet, eating too much of it can be dangerous. Statistics show that  most Americans eat too much salt. For your body to  serve  duly, you need to consume 500 mg a day.

What does sodium do?

It isn't mandatory to eradicate salt fully from your diet. Experts still recommend people use this for their bodies to serve duly.

Sodium is an element that balances body fluids, plays a part in muscle compression and relaxation, and transmits impulses. Too much sodium in your diet can have a negative effect on the body. This holds and draws in water, resulting in increased blood volume that makes your heart work harder than it used to.

Using herbs to lose weight

In this modern world, most of the foods on request are unhealthy. Because of this, you need to be smart about looking for foods that fit into your diet and produce weight loss results. However, adding fresh herbs to your dish can make all the difference, If you feel like you have the right  constituents.

There are tons of fresh herbs that you can use. Some of them include

parsley

basil

oregano

cumin

thyme

Rosemary

chives

Black pepper

nutmeg

cinnamon

peppers

chilli

Each of these can be salty or  spicy. There are several that are beautiful. Some herbs can be combined with fruits or foods for healthy spices and goodies that add flavor to your healthy diet. You can find them at your nearest local store.

First way in the use of fresh herbs
 Some people who are used to artificial foods may find it  grueling  to add these herbs to their foods,  thus getting started may be difficult with herbs, especially if you haven't considered this type of food for a long time. For you to be successful with these herbs, there are some tips to consider

Get fresh herbs.
The fresher the herbs, the higher the benefit. The dried herbs still have flavor but have no other health properties. However, simply chop them into small pieces and  also follow the instructions in your cookbook.

If you want to use fresh herbs.  Grow your own. Fresh herbs aren't as tough as some think.

However, start growing herbs in your garden , If you want to save and avoid the hassle of grocery shopping. This not only saves you time and money when buying groceries but also makes it much easier to cook your favorite recipes regularly.  It's a good idea to add fresh herbs to your diet, before you decide to add this, consult your doctor first. The reason is that some people are ill-disposed to some herbs. So, if you do not want any complications while losing weight, find out which herbs are good for you.

# Chapter Seventeen

## Change Your View about Whole Grains

A diet rich in whole grains can help combat belly bulge and reduce the risk of heart disease.

A new study showed that people who followed weight loss programs that included whole grain bread and cereals were more likely to successfully achieve their weight loss goals.

Additionally, those who considered a whole grain diet experienced a drop of about 38%

in CRP, or C-reactive protein, which is an indicator of inflammation in the body that is linked to heart disease.

The researchers said the results suggest that including whole grains in your weight loss plan may help you burn fat and reduce your risk of heart disease.

Whole Grains vs. Refined Grains

In a recent study, a group of overweight people with metabolic syndrome were divided into two groups. Metabolic syndrome is a collection of risk factors that increase the risk of diabetes and heart disease.

Both groups were advised to reduce calories

for a total of 12 weeks. However, one group was told to eat only whole grains  while the other was told not to eat whole grains.

In the end, both groups showed a succession of clients. Both have undergone a reduction in their body fat. However, people who belong to the group that only eats whole grains lost weight quickly. They also experienced other benefits. But people in the refined grains group received no other benefit.

Comprehensive sources

If you're looking for a whole-grain source, here are the different whole-grain products to consider:

full grain

oatmeal

Popcorn

Integral rice

whole corn


whole rye

darling

bulgur

triticale

Wild rice

buckwheat

whole barley

sorghum

andean millet


There are also whole grains like toasted
oats, popcorn, whole wheat snack chips, and
whole wheat flour that you can add to your

snacks or meals.

Whole grain products on food labels

When trying to find foods that contain
whole grains, choose foods with the
following characteristics:

bulgur
oatmeal
Integral rice
whole rye

whole oats
Wild rice
full grain
whole corn

When you come across labels like

"multigrain," "bran," "flour," "sifted grain," "100% wheat," etc., they usually don't contain whole grains.

You should keep in mind that colour is not the basis of whole grains. Some bread can be browned because of their ingredients or molasses. If you want to be sure, you should look at the nutritional facts.

# Chapter Eighteen

# Don't Forget The Water

There are several reasons why it is important to drink water while losing weight. Therefore, do not forget to drink water, as it can help you achieve all your weight loss goals.

Reasons why you should not forget water to lose weight

One of the main reasons you need to drink water while dieting is that it can help you avoid dehydration. The initial weight loss is caused by the loss of water. You should drink an adequate amount of water to stay hydrated.

The process of burning fat and calories also requires adequate water intake to keep you working efficiently. You have to remember that dehydration reduces the fat-burning process. Once you've burned calories, you create toxins like an exhaust pipe coming out of your car. Because of this, water plays an important role in removing toxins from your body.

If you're trying to lose weight to build abs and muscles, water helps maintain muscle tone by helping muscles contract and this lubricates joints. With proper hydration, you can reduce muscle and joint pain during exercise.

Many people know that healthy weight loss is related to getting a good amount of fibre. But without water, your weight loss will never be successful because you may suffer from constipation...

# Chapter Nineteen

# Use Affirmations To Stay On Course

Affirmations can help you get started. That's why it's important to use affirmations to keep you on track. Through these, it is possible to achieve all your weight loss goals. All you need is to be clear about what affirmations are and what they can do to make you effective in losing weight.

Definite statements

Affirmations are simply whatever you think

or say. People are constantly reinforcing what they want out of life with their beliefs and thoughts. For example, if you think losing weight is impossible and difficult, it will be. But once you believe that it may be difficult but you can achieve it, then it certainly will be. You must remember that actions follow thoughts. So with positive affirmations, your actions will also be positive, allowing you to keep moving forward.

Staying in the course is never an easy task, especially when you are surrounded by temptations. That is why affirmations are useful. Here are some of them:

I will follow a healthy and balanced diet.
I will follow a specific diet that will improve

my ability to lose extra pounds.

# Chapter Twenty

# The Benefits Of Maintaining A Healthy Weight

There are many advantages of loosing and maintaining a healthy weight. It not only improves the quality of life but also increases the quantity of life.

Here are the key benefits of maintaining a healthy weight:

Discomfort relief

Carrying extra pounds also affects someone's active lifestyle. Even a 5-10% weight loss will help alleviate various aches and pains associated with inactivity.

Extra pounds on your body can put more stress on your bones, muscles, and joints, causing them to work harder than normal just to move. However, by weighing less, your body can function efficiently and prevent damage that can prevent a person from successfully performing daily activities.

Healthier heart

If your weight is heavy, your heart may not be able to work effectively even when you are resting. However, if you maintain a healthy weight, you will increase the amount of blood going to various vital organs in your body, which will also allow your heart to do its job efficiently.

Maintaining a healthy weight also reduces the workload on the heart, which reduces the risk of heart attack, angina, and high blood pressure.

Lower risk of diabetes

According to some research and studies, obese people have a higher risk of developing type II diabetes. If you've already been diagnosed with this condition, it's important to lose weight, as this will give you better control. If you don't have this condition, maintaining a healthy weight reduces your risk of diabetes.

Cancer prevention

Experts said that weight loss plays an important role in the fight against cancer. Weight loss not only prevents the development of cancer but can also reduce the likelihood of developing several types of cancer known today. According to some studies, obese women are more likely to develop cancer of the gallbladder, breast, uterus, colon, cervix, and ovary, while obese men may develop prostate, rectal, and colon cancer.

Prevent osteoarthritis

Osteoarthritis is a disease in which patients experience joint pain. Being overweight could put many people at risk of developing this condition. However, with a healthy weight, this disorder can be easily prevented before it occurs.

Along with exercise and a healthy diet, the body's joints support less weight and prevent damage over time.

These are just a few of the many benefits of a healthy weight. So if you want to live healthier and bypass some diseases thereafter, now is the right time to start losing weight.

Recognizing the consequences isn't just a risk or problem that might force you to stop trying; It is also a positive factor that will drive you forward. You will never know the result if you only anticipate it; You should try to at least take a considerable amount of time. As long as you are acting you will never feel guilty because you have never tried and practised and you will no longer achieve the real results of your plans.

The rewards are achievable and can always be performed in the best possible way. Hard work deserves recognition, so start living healthy and in no time you will be satisfied with the results of happiness.

To Wrap It Up

Setting realistic weight loss goals is critical to leading a healthy lifestyle. If you want the effects of your hard work to last, you must follow the advice in this book. Keep in mind that you may not see results right away, but with time and effort, you're sure to be satisfied. I hope this information has been useful and helpful to you, good luck in your expedition to a successful weight loss and weight maintenance...

* 9 7 9 8 3 7 8 5 7 1 3 6 9 *